MW00835481

THE EDUCATED

A f

HOSPICE NURSE!!!

The Ultimate Hospice guide!!!

CREATED BY
MAKHAELA WILLIAMS, RN
OWNER OF HOSPICE NURSE BASICS

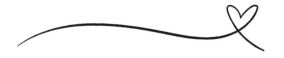

Medical Disclaimer

The information presented throughout this Book/EBOOK, *The Educated AF Hospice Nurse*, does not constitute any medical advice. This information does not override Medicare regulations, CMS guidelines, or any other federal law. This information is based on personal experiences and personal opinions.

Please seek advice from a licensed healthcare provider or your doctor for any particular health concerns before changing your healthcare routine or relying on this information presented, as these are just my personal opinions.

Copyright © [2024] by [MaKhaela Williams]

All rights reserved. No part of this ebook/book may be reproduced or transmitted in any form or by any means, electronic or mechanical, including photocopying, recording or by any information storage and retrieval system, or AI without permission in writing from the copyright holder MaKhaela Williams.

This is a work of fiction. Names, characters, places and incidents either are the product of the author's imagination or are used fictitiously, and any resemblance to actual persons, living or dead, businesses, companies, events or locales is entirely coincidental.

Published by [MaKhaela Williams]

BY MAKHAELA WILLIAMS
HOSPICE NURSE BASICS

HOSPICENURSEBASICS@GMAIL.COM

THE EDUCATED AF HOSPICE NURSE!!

ABOUT THE AUTHOR

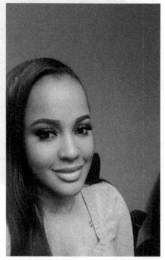

MaKhaela Williams, RN

Being a nurse is a challenging yet rewarding profession. I knew I wanted to be a nurse since I was five (it was my favorite card in the OLD MAID deck—haha, showing my age!).

As a nurse today, I am honored that I followed my dreams. I can't think of any other profession that is more fulfilling, and I have worked in the healthcare field for almost 20 years... (Now that's crazy AF!!!) I guess it's true that time flies when you enjoy what you do.

I knew that becoming a hospice nurse was my calling. I remember my first encounter with losing a patient as a CNA and how caring and comforting her hospice team was to her and her family. I then had a personal experience with hospice care, and from that point on, I knew I wanted to be a hospice nurse.

A career as a hospice nurse is awesome! You meet so many different people from different cultures and backgrounds, and I can't think of a more rewarding career.

4.

6.

Contents

Contents

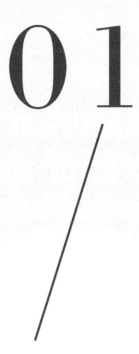

01

CHAPTER 1
Introduction

01

INTRODUCTION

ONE OF THE ESSENTIAL ASPECTS OF BEING NOT ONLY A HOSPICE NURSE, BUT A HEALTHCARE PROFESSIONAL IS **DOCUMENTATION.**

We spend so much time taking care of our patients and documenting that we often neglect ourselves. If not done efficiently, charting can become a burden and disturb our work-life balance.

It's not fair to ourselves or to our loved ones to spend so much time in front of the computer documenting and not enjoying our lives. In this book, I'm going to provide you with the valuable tools needed to improve your charting skills and enhance overall charting your efficiency. This book features ways to:

1. Provide work-life balance.
2. Spend less time documenting.
3. Document more efficiently.
4. Ability to document in real time.
5. Charting specifics to the diagnosis.
6. Improve patient care.

Watch your life become balanced AF by implementing
The Educated AF Hospice Nurse Guide.

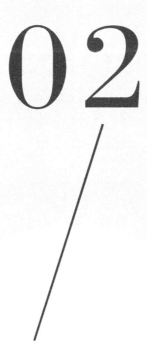

02

CHAPTER 1
Documentation Best Practices

02

DOCUMENTATION BEST PRACTICES!!!!

I KNOW WE HEAR IT OVER AND OVER AGAIN, BUT TRUST ME, IT WORKS. DOCUMENT AT THE BEDSIDE AS MUCH AS POSSIBLE!!!

Most EMR systems are primarily just pushing buttons and doing a narrative at the end. Once you get to know that EMR system, you should be able to zoom right through your visit notes.

Document in real-time during those more flexible visits. If you have extra time, spend that time charting. You can even chart in your car. This, along with my other tips listed below, will guarantee that you will become more efficient and spend less time charting at home. Who wants to do that? WTF!

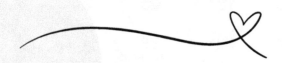

MY TOP 10

DOCUMENTATION BEST PRACTICES!!!!

1. For every patient on your caseload, create your **Patient Cheat Sheet** (example/ template in Chapter 3)

2. **Be specific, clear, and concise.** You don't need the fluff when charting, trust me.

3. **Communicate with patients and families!!** When you create a schedule for your patients and families, make sure to tell them it is tentative because emergencies happen. That way, on those crazy days, you don't feel forced to see everyone, and everyone has that mutual understanding.

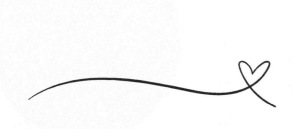

DOCUMENTATION BEST PRACTICES!!!!

4. **Communicate with your coworkers and supervisors.** You will be surprised how important this is. There could be a nurse that is having a light day, that may be willing to help you when you're in a bind. Let's spread the love!

5. **One comprehensive visit per week per patient.** The rest are Follow-up Visits. There should be no more than three comprehensive visits a day. Break it up! There is no rule that the first visit of the week has to be a comprehensive visit, and if you do one weekly, you will never miss the every 14-day regulation.

6. **Be objective and chart what you observe.** For example, Paint the Picture: The patient reports pain, eats a percentage of the meal, sits in a reclined position, etc. (See Chapter 4 for great tips!)

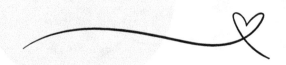

DOCUMENTATION BEST PRACTICES!!!!

7. Use a nursing format when charting. I like the **SOAP** format:

- **Subject**-concern, complaint, change.
- **Observe**-labs, vitals, exams, diagnostics, and what you see.
- **Assess**-S+O=Assess (What is the problem?)
- **Plan**-New orders, med changes, how do we fix the problem?

8. **Add pertinent changes to your patient cheat sheet** so you remember to mention those topics in your IDT/Recert note. COPY and PASTE from the cheat sheet into the IDT/Recert Note and/or visit note.

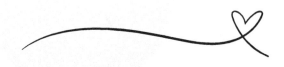

DOCUMENTATION BEST PRACTICES!!!!

9. **Week of IDT and RECERTS:** Do what I call a RECERT VISIT or IDT VISIT. The narrative written in your weekly Nurse Note during your nurse visit, should also be used as your IDT/RECERT NOTE as well. Yes, that means COPY and PASTE your note and change the First sentence.

*Visit Note -"RN Visit made to assess the patient for recertification/IDT...."

*IDT/Recert Note: "As discussed in RN Visit Note, the patient was assessed for Recertification/IDT."
USE THE SAME NOTE...it will save you so much time

10. **Use your Hospice Nurse Basics Paint the Picture guide and LCDs** while charting. Upload them to your computer or email. This will ensure that you are documenting to the negative and to the hospice diagnosis.

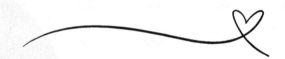

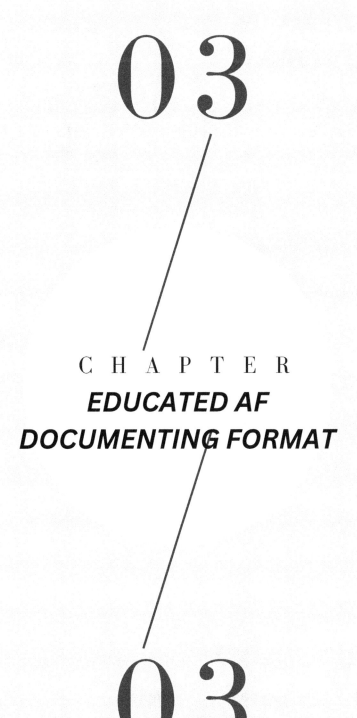

03

C H A P T E R
EDUCATED AF
DOCUMENTING FORMAT

03

PATIENT CHEAT SHEET!!!

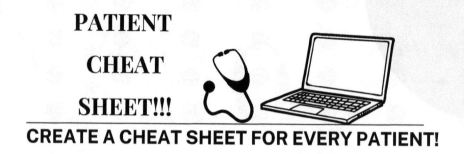

CREATE A CHEAT SHEET FOR EVERY PATIENT!

EXAMPLE CHEAT SHEET

Patient Name:

Patient Caregiver/Facility Name:

Patient Address and phone number:

Gender:

Patient Age and DOB:

Hospice Dx:

Co-morbidities: (unrelated and related)

Cert Period:

Attending Physician:

Goals for next 2 weeks:

Notes: **(see next page for example)**

PATIENT CHEAT SHEET!!!

CREATE A CHEAT SHEET FOR EVERY PATIENT!

Add all pertinent information to notes-falls, weight loss, infections, symptoms, caregiver info, level of care changes, comparative data (See Chapter 5), etc...ANYTHING!

EXAMPLE CHEAT SHEET NOTES

1/1/24-Patient had a non-injury fall

1/24/24-Bowel regimen Senna S 1 tab PO BID Initiated

02/7/24-16f, 10cc Foley catheter changed

03/01/24-Patient weighs 112lbs.

03/04/24-Patient moved to named facility for respite

03/31/24-New order for Lasix 20mg PO daily for fluid retention

04/01/24-Patient weighs 108lbs.

IMPORTANT!!!: Keep a running tab of your cheat sheet notes for each patient, and never delete these notes. This information creates the best comparative notes that can be used in your recert and IDT Notes

PATIENT
CHEAT
SHEET!!!

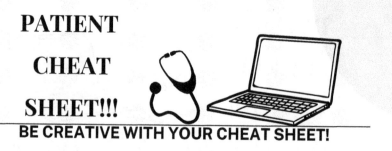

BE CREATIVE WITH YOUR CHEAT SHEET!

-You can add anything that you feel is important to your cheat sheet.

-For example, I like to put if the patient is diabetic or has a thyroid issue or any endocrine condition because I always forget that when it comes time to chart, LOL!!!

Put the CHEAT SHEET information into a paragraph for your IDT and Recert Notes. This will save a ton of time!

EXAMPLE IDT NOTE:

Mary Doe is an 88-year-old female with a hospice diagnosis of CHF with comorbidities of atherosclerosis and hypoxia. She resides in assisted living. Her current cert period is 60-4. Her attending physician is Dr. Jane. Over the last two weeks (insert nursing notes/comparative data) (See Chapter 5 for an example recert note). Goals for the next two weeks.

Keep this document in your work email, where it's secure, so you can copy and paste it. This will save you a ton of time on charting.

ADMISSION NOTE

My Admit Note is Three Parts/Paragraphs:

Part one:

- Patient's age
- Gender
- Primary Hospice Diagnosis
- Secondary Hospice Diagnosis
- Related Co-morbidities
- Unrelated Co-morbidities
- Smoker/Non-smoker-(Medical Director needs this information for certification)
- Patient choice for Attending Physician

Part One Example:

Patient is a 91-year-old female with a primary hospice diagnosis of Alzheimer's and a secondary diagnosis of severe protein-calorie malnutrition. Patient has related co-morbidities of abnormal weight loss, debility, anxiety, dysphagia, B12 deficiency, fatigue, and constipation. Patient has unrelated comorbidities of hypothyroidism, hypertension, dementia, and macular degeneration. Patient has a history of smoking but quit 20 years ago. Patient's attending physician is Dr. Jane Doe.

ADMISSION NOTE

Part two:

Hospice...Why now?/ Paint the Picture/ Review all records/ CREATE COMPARATIVE DATA:

- Residence and Caregivers

- Disease onset/condition duration /response or lack of response to treatment

- Alertness and orientation/Disorientation

- Cognitive changes- (agitation, restlessness, anxiety, orientation to place, time, self, delusions)

- PPS, FAST, NYHA Scale

- Pertinent vitals, weight, MAC, BMI

- Pertinent labs and diagnostics

- Degree of frailty/time-to-task completion)-USE COMPARATIVE DATA (See Chapter 5)

- Diagnosis specifics-refer to S/Sx r/t primary and secondary dx-Disease specific information per the local coverage determinations (LCDs)

- Related Co-morbidities

- ·Deterioration of functional abilities- dependence on ADLs

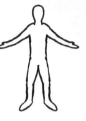

Body Systems:

1. **Integumentary**-skin breakdown, wounds, nails, ulcers
2. **Skeletal**-fractures, falls, surgeries, transfers, assistive devices
3. **Muscular**-pain, ambulation status, ambulation devices
4. **Nervous**-speech changes, hours of sleep, vision, fever, and pain
5. **Endocrine**-thyroid, diabetes, hormonal disorder
6. **Cardiovascular**-blood, cardiac, edema, circulation
7. **Lymphatic**-Edema
8. **Digestive**-Food and water intake and output, dietary needs, changes in stools, NPO, puree, thickened liquids, weight changes, dysphagia
9. **Urinary**-incontinence, UTI, catheter, infections, changes in urine output, kidney failure
10. **Respiratory**-SOA, pneumonia, infections, oxygen
11. **Reproductive**-male and female reproductive
12. **Immune**-white blood count, risk of infection

ADMISSION NOTE

Part Two Example:

Patient resting comfortably in a recliner located in her bedroom upon arrival. *(Residence and caregivers)* She resides in a lockdown memory care unit, where she receives around-the-clock nursing care. *(Disease Onset)* Patient was dx with Alzheimer's in May 2019, and despite usage of medications, including Namenda and Aricept, the patient's condition continues to progress *(lack of response to treatment)*. *(Alertness and Orientation)* Patient is alert and oriented to self only. Disoriented to event, time, and place. She is agitated with care and has frequent moments of delusions that are being managed with Seroquel 25mg PO BID. *(Scales)* FAST 7D PPS 40%. *(Secondary diagnosis)* Her current weight was 108 lbs. 4 months ago, the patient weighed 120 lbs, causing a 10% weight loss over the last 4 months, and she has a BMI of 13. LMAC14. *(Labs)* Has a serum albumin 2.0 on 03/01/2021. Speech is garbled and only speaks 5 words or less. *(Comorbidities, LCD's)*One year ago, she was able to speak 3-word sentences. Speech and mobility continued to decline despite therapy attempts. She is unable to ambulate and has a chair or bed-bound existence, spending 24 hours a day in bed, Broda chair, or reclining chair. Transfers with Hoyer lift and assist x2. *(ADL's)* Dependent on others for bathing, dressing, toileting, and hand-fed during meals.....

ADMISSION NOTE CONT...

Part three:

- Trajectory of diagnosis
- Services provided
- Hospice Level of Care
- Disciplines
- Visit Frequencies DME ordered
- Comfort Kit orders
- Hospice binder and contact information

Part 3 Example:

Dr. Yarn has referred the patient to hospice as her trajectory of illness supports the six-month prognosis. Despite dialysis 3x a week, her disease continues to progress. Patient and family have chosen hospice services to receive assistance with end-of-life education and support as disease progresses, medication and symptom management, pain management, fall, and safety prevention teachings, skin breakdown prevention, and supplemental oxygen education. Family and patient have requested no further hospitalizations and to receive palliative measures only. Patient admitting hospice level of care is Routine Home Care. The following hospice services will be provided: Nursing visits 2x a week, HHA 2x a week, Initial Chaplain visit, Initial Medical Social Worker visit, and volunteer has been requested. DME, including oxygen concentrator 5LPM, 2 E-tanks, nebulizer machine, hospital bed with LAL mattress, and bedside commode, have been ordered. Morphine comfort kit reviewed with patient and daughter, Kim Doe. Hospice binder was reviewed and left in patient's bedroom. Hospice hours and contact information reviewed.

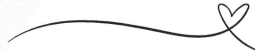

Items that require orders at Admission:

- Wounds
- Drains
- Falls
- Diet
- Infections
- DME
- Comfort Kit/ Medication orders
- Standing orders
- Hospital orders

DEATH VISIT NOTE

The nice thing about writing a death note is that most EMR systems have become very detailed with death notes, and typically, only a small narrative is required once documentation is completed.

When creating your Death Note, **CHART TO THE EXCEPTION.** You shouldn't be repetitive with your note. Simply paint a picture and describe your assessment.

If your EMR does not ask for the below information, please include it in the narrative:

- Medication Disposal procedure
- Medical Attachments (colostomy, catheter, etc.)
- Funeral Home Name
- Time body was released to the Funeral Home
- Location of death (home or facility name)
- Level of care- (Routine, Respite, Inpatient, or Continuous)
- Time MD, DME, Pharmacy, Hospice team, etc. were contacted
- Belongings (jewelry, clothing, watches, etc.)
- State Coroner/Medical Examiner Reports

DEATH VISIT NOTE

Death Note Narrative Example

Patient is an 89-year-old male admitted to hospice services on 11/16/2023 with a primary hospice diagnosis of Alzheimer's Disease with a secondary diagnosis of Protein Calorie Malnutrition. On 01/01/2024 at 0415 a.m. I received a call from facility nurse Stacey Doe, stating that the patient was found unresponsive in his hospital bed at 0400 a.m. On-call nurse visit made. Arrived at named facility at 0500 a.m. Patient is non-responsive in a hospital bed, lying in the supine position. Patient is without an apical or peripheral pulse. He has no blood pressure or respirations. He has no response to stimulation, and pupils are fixed and non-responsive. The patient is without heart and lung sounds. The patient's time of death is 0505 a.m. (make sure the time of death is at least five minutes after your assessment). Patient's son, Jon Doe, is at the bedside and grieving appropriately. According to the son, the patient was last seen breathing at 0350 a.m. and had a peaceful passing. The attending physician, Dr. Jane Doe, was notified at 0510 a.m. Funeral home of choice was contacted at 0515 a.m. Postmortem care provided with standard precautions. Medications are destroyed per facility protocol. The named funeral home arrived at the facility at 0600 a.m., and the body was released at 0610 a.m. Staff and family grieving appropriately. Bereavement services have been explained to the patient's son, who is also the patient's primary contact.

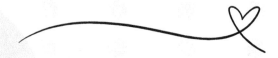

IMPORTANT!!!: Keep a running tab of your cheat sheet notes for each patient, and never delete these notes.

Modify when needed.

This information creates the best comparative notes that can be used in your recert and IDT Notes

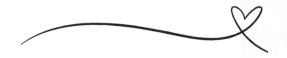

RECERT NOTE

Always compare and contrast from your last RECERT and/or IDT NOTE for the most accurate information and comparative data.

This information will be easily found on your running tab.

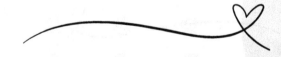

Recert Note Example

Patient Name , Age, and Gender: _____

Diagnosis _____

Co-morbidities _____

Code Status: _____

Cert Period: _____

Attending Physician: _____

Pertinent Medical History: _____

Pain level: 0 1 2 3 4 5 6 7 8 9 10   Pain medication:

Supporting Disease Data/Trajectory:_____

PPS, NYHA, and/or FAST score: _____

MAC, Weight, or BMI Changes:_____

Any new doctor appts or exams: _____

Careplan updates/Medication changes:_____

Wounds, infections, incidents:_____

DME ordered: _____

New Labs:_____

Spiritual/Psychosocial Needs: _____

Pertinent Needs (respite, funeral plans, DNR, etc):_____

Education:_____

Visit Frequency for every IDT mem: _____

Goals over the next 2 weeks/follow-ups: _____

EXAMPLE NOTE/PARAGRAPH

Mary Doe is an 88-year-old female with a hospice dx of CHF with co morbs of atherosclerosis and hypoxia. She resides in assisted living. Current cert period 60-4 and has a DNR code status. Her attending physician is Dr. Jane. Over the last two weeks (*insert nursing notes/recert notes/comparative data (See Chapter 3 and Chapter 5).*

RESPITE NOTE

- Transportation and time of arrival
- Respite facility name and length of stay
- Facility contact name and building codes
- Ensure facility has hospice contact number and binder
- Ensure contracts between facility and hospice are completed
- Make sure patient's room number is correct in the chart
- Ensure patient has all belongings-clothing and supplies
- Review medications and orders with staff
- Review DME
- Any changes in condition/pertinent infomation
- Update family and IDT with visit findings

Respite Note Example:

RN respite visit. Patient was transported to Named Nursing and Rehab today at 0915 a.m. via medical transportation. She arrived at the facility at 1000 a.m. for a five-day respite stay. Patient is currently sleeping in a hospital bed upon arrival. Patient assigned room number has been updated in the system, along with door code to enter the building after hours. Spoke to ADON Jackie, who informed me that all paperwork has been completed, and no additional documents are needed at this time. Medications and wound care orders reviewed with Nurse Jackie. Pharmacy has delivered all medications and DME, including wheelchair, and hospital bed was delivered prior to patient's arrival. Foam dressings, wound cleanser, zinc barrier cream, large briefs, wipes, chux, and medium gloves delivered and left in the patient's closet. Hospice binder left at nursing station. Staff given tentative hospice disciplines schedule and hospice contact phone number. Called patient's son and informed him that patient is adjusting well to respite stay and that a member from hospice will visit her daily.

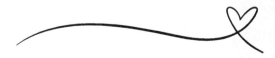

CONTINUOUS CARE NOTE

When conducting vigil visit or sitting continuous care, you want to chart hourly and PRN. Make sure you chart every intervention. If it's not charted, it didn't happen. Here's an example....

0700 a.m.-bed bath performed. Linens changed. Patient tolerated well.

0800 a.m.-BP 78/59 P41 T98.0 R12 O2 85%RA

0845 a.m.-Patient turned onto the left side. Pain at 7 via FACES scale. Moans and grimaces. Administer Morphine 0.5mL SL. Medication control sheet updated.

0900 a.m.-BP P R T O2

0930 a.m.- Audible secretions noted. Lungs assessed. Administered Hyoscyamine 0.125mg SL

0945 a.m.-Patient turned onto the right side. Pain at 7 via FACES scale. Moans and grimaces. Administer Morphine 0.5mL SL Medication controlled sheet updated.

1000 a.m.-BP P R T O2

1030 a.m.- Patient soiled with small BM. Peri care performed.Patient turned onto the left side. Pain at 8 via FACES scale. Moans, frowns, and grimaces. Administer Morphine 0.5mL SL. Medication control sheet updated.

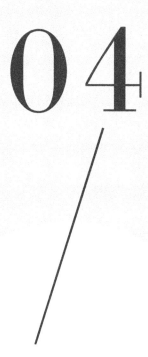

04

C H A P T E R
Painting the Picture

04

Heart
Failure

Paint the Picture

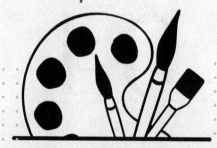

Heart Failure

1. Severe/extreme distressing fatigue and weakness

2. Chair or home existence/sleeps in recliner or hospital bed

3. Oxygen dependence at night, as needed, or continuously.

4. Shortness of breath at rest, speaking, eating, exertion or rapid and shallow breathing

5. Poor gait and posture/uses assistive devices

6. Swelling/peripheral edema in the legs, ankles, abdomen, feet, face, etc..

7. Inability to perform ADLS-peri-care, bathing, eating, swallowing, feeding, transfers, toilet hygiene, dressing

8. Irregular or rapid heartbeat (arrhythmias)

9. Chest pain or discomfort

10. Difficulty sleeping or staying asleep/sleeps with HOB elevated or in upright position

Heart Failure

11. Increased urination at night

12. Classifies as an IV on the NYHA scale

13. Loss of appetite and unintentional weight loss

14. Confusion or disorientation

15. Anxiety, agitation, or restlessness

16. Pallor or coolness of the skin, specifically in the hands and feet, tingliness or neuropathy

17. Ejection fraction 20% or less

18. Hx of cardiac arrest. MI, CVA

19. Coughing, wheezing, or gurgling sounds during breathing/impaired lung sounds

20. Poor response/changes to medications-diuretics and vasodilators

Heart Failure

S: Patient feeling short of breath and breathing is labored.
O: Oxygen saturation level is 90% on room air, 1+ abdominal edema.
A: Patient in fluid overload.
P: Administer diuretics, PRN Oxygen, and nebulizer treatment.

S: Patient reports swelling in the legs and ankles.
O: 2+Edema in bilateral lower extremities.
A: Patient has peripheral edema.
P: Patient encouraged to elevate BLE, compression hose ordered, and review s/sx worsening edema with patient and family.

S: Patient confused regarding medications over the weekend.
O: Patient's blood pressure 191/101.
A: Patient is hypertensive due to not taking prescibed medications.
 P: Administer blood pressure and diuretic as ordered. Monitor for effectiveness. Set up weekly pill organizer.

S: Patient reports trouble sleeping and restlessness.
O: Patient prefers to sleep in recliner.
A: Patient has insomnia r/t heart failure symptoms of dyspnea.
P: Obtained order for hospital bed with low air loss mattress and Melatonin gummies 5 mg Qhs.

Alzheimer's/ Dementia

Paint the Picture

Alzheimer's/Dementia

1. Inability to make needs known, communicate verbally or understand language

2. Dysphagia/hx or risk of aspiration

3. Low albumin less than 2.5

4. Severe memory loss, including forgetting family members and friends

5. Inability to perform basic activities of daily living, such as dressing, transfers, eating, and bathing-total care

6. Difficulty walking or standing, often confined to a bed or wheelchair

7. Weight loss or cachexia (muscle wasting)/contractures/foot drop

8. Recurrent infections or frequent antibiotic usage

9. Increased sleeping and decreased wakefulness

10. Limited response to stimuli or surroundings

Alzheimer's/Dementia

11. Skin breakdown or pressure ulcers/bony prominences

12. Loss of facial expressions and emotional responses

13. Thickened liquids/soft foods or other dietary changes

14. Changes in vital signs, such as heart rate and blood pressure

15. Increased confusion, disorientation, and agitation, particularly in the late afternoon and evening (known as "sundowning")

16. Poor hygiene/incontinence

17. Changes in personality-outburst and mood swings, violent behavior

18. Wandering/elopement risk

19. Impaired judgement

20. Pocket food

Alzheimer's/Dementia

S: Patient is verbally aggressive toward staff.
O: Patient is pacing and making threatening statements.
A: Behavioral disturbance.
P: Implement de-escalation techniques and administer prescribed PRN medication as needed.

S: Patient was found wandering in the hallway.
O: Patient is disoriented and unable to provide current location.
A: Increased risk of falls and elopement.
P: Implement fall prevention measures and monitor patient closely for safety precautions.

S: Patient is refusing to take medication.
O: Patient is unable to identify medications and appears anxious.
A: Difficulty with medication management.
P: Provide medication education and simplify medication regimen as appropriate.

S: Patient experienced a fall in the bathroom.
O: Patient reports pain in left hip. X-ray shows no fracture.
A: Increased risk of falls and injury.
P: Initiate fall prevention measures and monitor for signs of pain or injury.

Cancer

Paint the Picture

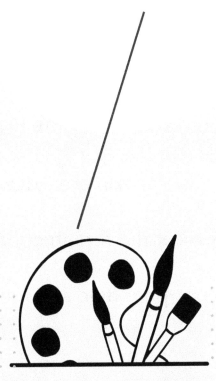

Cancer

1. Extreme/distressing fatigue and weakness-poor stamina and endurance, tires easily.

2. Changes in skin color-jaundice, ashen, cyanotic, pale, etc.

3. Chronic, severe pain that can be hard to manage

4. Cognitive changes-Delirium, hallucinations, agitation, etc.

5. Difficulty with ADLs-with or without assist

6. Shortness of air, difficulty breathing

7. Nausea, vomiting, dry heaves

8. Risk for skin breakdown

9. Hx or risk for infection

10. Anorexia-poor fluid and food intake

Cancer

11. Risk for bleed/bleeding precaution

12. Fluid retention-brain, lungs, ascites, etc.

13. Weight Loss

14. Sores/ulcers-mouth or pressure sores

15. Changes in sleep pattern

16. Malnutrition-poor appetite

17. Peripheral edema/neuropathy

18. Comatose/Vegetative state/Encephalopathy

19. Social Isolation

20. Cachexia or frailty/
use of assistive devices

Cancer

S: Patient reports bruising on her arms and legs.
O: Several new areas of bruising noted on upper extremities with no signs or reports of trauma.
A: Bruising is due to prescribed blood thinner.
P: Initiate bleeding precautions. Medication education.

S: Patient's spouse reports the patient states there are children running in room.
O: Patient smiling and laughing while hallucinating.
A: Patient experiencing delirium without behavioral disturbances.
P: Monitor and review s/sx of distress with spouse and educate on disease process.

S: Patient's wife reports shallow breathing, no food intake for a week, and patient continues to be non-responsive to stimulation.
O: Patient resting comfortably, O2 86% on 3LPM, BP60/49 HR41.
A: Patient is actively dying.
P: Monitor and educate on s/sx of impending death. Inform IDT and request visit from chaplain and social worker.

Debility

Paint the Picture

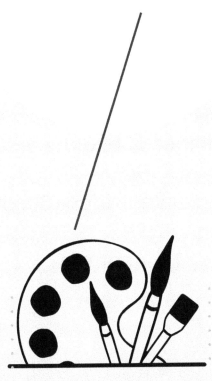

Debility

1. Severe weakness and fatigue

2. Poor stamina and endurance

3. Poor gait and posture/contractures/foot drop

4. Poor caloric intake

5. Dehydration/poor capillary refills

6. Bed/chairbound

7. Difficulty swallowing

8. Incontinence of bladder and bowel

9. Protein malnutrition (Chapter 4)

10. Anorexia

Debility

11. Difficulty breathing

12. Pain

13. Loss of muscle mass/weight loss

14. Recurring infections

15. Poor urine output

16. Constipation

17. Hypotensive

18. Cognitive decline-loss of interests

19. Risk for skin breakdown/wounds/poor skin integrity/bony prominences

20. Changes in consciousness

Debility

S: Patient's daughter reports that the patient has been in bed for over a week.
O: Patient is increasingly weak and fatigued.
A: Patient is debilitated and declining clinically.
P: Hospital bed with low air loss mattress ordered.

S: Patient reports abdominal pain and discomfort.
O: Last reported BM was four days ago; bowel sounds are hypoactive.
A: Patient is constipated.
P: Encourage high-fiber diet; administer PRN stool softeners.

S: Patient is weak and unable to bear weight.
O: Patient is unable to assist with transfers.
A:Loss of muscle mass with joint pain in BUE.
P: Ordered Hoyer lift for transfers and initiated pain regimen.

S: Patient reports burning while urinating.
O: Patient positive for three UTIs in six weeks.
A: Recurring infections.
P: New order for prophylactic antibiotics and cranberry tabs. UIT prevention education provided.

Renal Failure

Paint the Picture

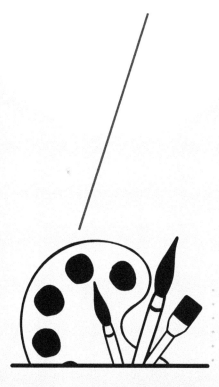

Renal Failure

1. Tires easily/chronic fatigue

2. Poor appetite

3. Chronic nausea and vomiting

4. Changes in sleep pattern

5. Shortness of breath/ supplemental oxygen use

6. Fluid retention/overload/ascites/edema

7. Pruritis/ itchy skin

8. Altered mental state: confusion, agitation, etc.

9. Muscle cramps/ tingling and numbness

10. Hypertensive

Renal Failure

11. Cold or Heat intolerance

12. Poor response to diuretics

13. Poor skin integrity/bruises easily/discoloration/rashes

14. High risk for infections

15. Poor urine output-less than 400cc a day

16. Serum Creatinine above 8.0

17. Neuropathy/use of assistive devices

18. Changes in bladder habits-blood in urine, odor, scant, urgency, etc...

19. Hyperkalemic

20. Poor caloric intake

Renal Failure

S: Patient reports pain in her legs rated at a 7/10 and describes the pain as cramps.
O: Legs are red in color with 3+ edema BLE.
A: Fluid overload causing leg cramps and discomfort.
P: Order obtained for compression hose. Patient encouraged to elevate BLE. Initiate pain regimen.

S: Patient's spouse reports blood in urine with an odor.
O: Patient is increasingly confused and has a fever of 100.9 temporal.
A: Patient showing s/sx of possible UTI.
P: Order obtained for stat UA. Initiate pain regimen for pain and fever.

S: Caregiver reports patient will not wake up for lunch.
O: Caregiver is attempting to feed the patient while she is weak and fatigued.
A: Force feeding and force drinking.
P: Review disease process with patient caregiver. Review the importance of comfort meals along with the importance of not force-feeding and its side effects.

Liver Failure

Paint the Picture

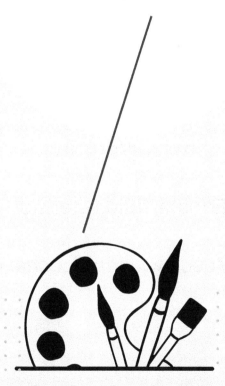

Liver Failure

1. Jaundice/ashen discoloration

2. Ascites/abnormal abdominal girth

3. Fatigue/poor endurance

4. Nausea and vomiting

5. Loss of appetite/anorexia

6. Cognitive changes/Encephalopathy

7. Bleeding risk/bruise easily

8. Itching/pruritus

9. Edema/fluid retention

10. Muscle wasting/cachexia

Liver Failure

11. Shortness of breath

12. Sleep disturbances

13. Dietary changes/ malnutrition

14. Reduced urine output/s/sx of renal failure

15. Increased risk of infections

16. PT >5 seconds/INR> 1.5

17. PleurX Drain

18. Albumin <2.5

19. Hx of Hepatitis

20. Hx alcohol abuse

Liver Failure

S: Patient has severe abdominal pain.
O: Patient's skin is yellow/jaundice in color and abdominal girth increased by 3 cm since yesterday.
A: Expected findings of end-stage liver failure.
P: PRN pain med and drain ascites via PleurX.

S: Patient report SOA and chest pain.
O: BP 199/101, O2 89% RA, RR 23.
A: Patient in respiratory distress.
P: Administer PRN supplemental oxygen and PRN morphine.

S: Patient c/o sleep disturbances d/t itching.
O: Skin is dry and flaky with visible scratch marks in bilateral upper extremities.
A: Pruritus r/t liver failure.
P: Administer PRN Benadryl and instruct to moisturize skin daily and as needed.

S: Patient's wife reports no urine output for 36 hours.
O: Poor urine output, dry skin, poor skin turgor.
A: Dehydration.
P: Obtain order for straight catheterization. Monitor intake and output.

CVA/Stroke

Paint the Picture

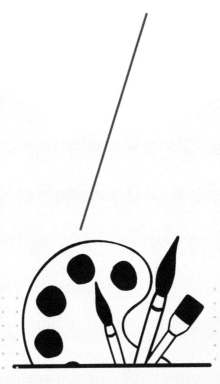

CVA/Stroke

1. Tingly, numbness, or weakness

2. Aphasia or impaired speech

3. Migraines/severe headaches

4. Poor vision-doubled, blurred, blindness, etc.

5. Feelings of vertigo and/or dizziness

6. Poor gait/use of assistive devices

7. Confusion/disorientation

8. Nausea and vomiting.

9. Has a history of convulsions/seizures

10. Body and/or facial paralysis or deformities

CVA/Stroke

11. Difficulty swallowing/hx of aspiration

12. Dependence on others for ADLs

13. Inability to control bowel or bladder function

14. Difficulty breathing or shortness of breath

15. Chest pain or palpitations

16. PPS lower than 40%

17. Hx of infections-respiratory, UTI, sepsis

18. Skeletomuscular contractures/tremors/involuntary muscle movements

19. Comatose/vegetative state/Encephalopathy

20. Malnutrition or albumin less than 2.5

CVA/Stroke

S: The patient's husband reports the patient chokes when swallowing water.
O: Patient coughing when taking small sips of fluid.
A: Patient experiencing residual side effect of dysphagia from CVA.
P: Obtain an order for speech therapy, thickened liquids, and soft foods.

S: Patient leans to left while sitting in wheelchair.
O: Patient is unable to change positions/turns.
A: Patient has right-sided paralysis
P: Educate on skin breakdown precautions and changing positions at least every two hours.

S: Patient communicates with dry-erase board.
O: Patient is unable to verbally make needs known.
A: Patient has aphasia.
P: Provide patient with proper tools for communication and inform Hospice IDT.

COPD/

Respiratory Failure

Paint the Picture

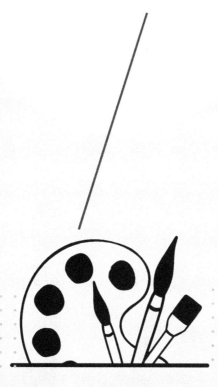

COPD/
Respiratory Failure

1. Severe shortness of breath, even when resting, speaking, eating, talking, and exertions

2. Chronic cough/ thick build-up

3. Decreased ability to cough up mucus/poor response to breathing medications

4. Rapid breathing

5. Wheezing or whistling sound when breathing/impaired lung sounds-crackles or diminished

6. Chest tightness or discomfort

7. Difficulty sleeping due to breathing problems

8. Extreme fatigue or weakness-poor stamina and endurance and tires easily

9. Loss of appetite

10. Unintentional weight loss of more than 10% in the last 6 months

COPD/
Respiratory Failure

11. Swelling in the ankles, feet, or legs

12. Bluish tint to the skin, lips, or nails (cyanosis)

13. Confusion or disorientation

14. Increased heart rate at above 100, even at rest

15. Uses supplemental oxygen PRN or continuously

16. O2 saturation at 88% or less on room air

17. Chronic steroid use

18. Thin extremities with a barrel chest

19. Poor skin integrity-thin/thick and calloused

20. Clubbed or discolored nails

COPD/
Respiratory Failure

S: Patient short of breath, congested, and increased coughing.
O: Oxygen saturation at 92% on 3 LPM, wheezing in LLL, productive cough with yellow-green sputum.
A: COPD exacerbation, s/sx of respiratory infections.
P: Administer nebulizer treatment and obtain order to increase oxygen rate and antibiotics

S: Patient is feeling weak and very fatigued.
O: Oxygen saturation drops to 84% from 93% on 4LPM of supplemental oxygen with exertions.
A: Increased urinary incontinence due to dyspnea.
P: Ordered a bedside commode.

S: Patient c/o feeling anxious and unable to breathe.
O: Oxygen saturation at 89% on room air with respirations at 26 BPM.
A: Patient in respiratory distress and anxiety.
P: Administer O2 via nasal cannula at 3LPM and PRN Lorazepam.

S: Patient reports feeling more short of breath and unable to catch her breath.
O: Vitals are WNL, oxygen saturation at 90% on room air, increased wheezing heard in RUL.
A: COPD exacerbation, patient had nebulizer treatment 30 mins ago.
P: Administer PRN morphine and supplemental oxygen, monitor oxygen saturation and respiratory effort, encourage deep breathing exercise

Parkinson's

Paint the Picture

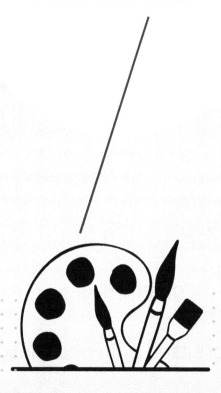

Parkinson's

1. Difficulty swallowing-coughing and choking/ hx or risk of aspiration

2. Blank stare

3. Severe tremors that interfere with daily activities/involuntary muscle movements

4. Increased rigidity/stiffness in muscles/contractures/foot drop

5. Significant loss of mobility and balance

6. Inability to perform activities of daily living, such as dressing, bathing, and grooming

7. Unable to make needs known

8. Hand-fed by others

9. Shuffled gait

10. Increased pain and discomfort

Parkinson's

11. Muffled or garbled speech

12. Unable to sit in the upright position/use of assistive devices-wheel chair, Broda, cushions, etc.

13. Low albumin-malnutrition

14. Skin breakdown or at risk

15. Mouth drooling

16. Shortness of breath/oxygen use/reduced lung sounds

17. S/sx of dementia (Chapter 4)

18. Recurrent infections, such as pneumonia or urinary tract infections

19. Poor stamina and endurance

20. Dietary changes-thickened liquids, soft foods, etc.

Parkinson's

S: The patient's wife reports difficulty swallowing when drinking liquids.
O: Patient coughing when drinking apple juice.
A: Parkinson's has caused worsening dysphagia.
P: Obtain an order for nectar thick liquids

S: The patient reports difficulty breathing.
O: Oxygen saturation is 89% on room air.
A: Parkinson's has caused decreased lung capacity.
P: Obtain an order for supplemental oxygen.

S: Patient reports feelings of depression.
O: The patient was tearful during nurse visit.
A: Patient concerned about who will make medical decisions for them if they are unable to make their own decisions.
P: Consult with Hospice SW for assistance with Advance Directive paperwork.

S: Staff reports difficulty sleeping and wandering at night.
O: The patient is fatigued often during the day hours.
A: Parkinson's disease has affected the patient's sleep pattern.
P: Order obtain for Seroquel 25mg Qhs and a wander alarm bracelet.

Protein-Calorie Malnutrition

Paint the Picture

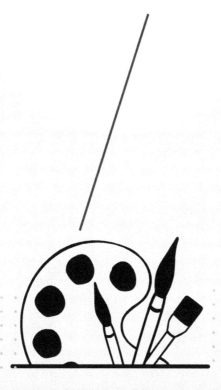

Protein-Calorie Malnutrition

1. 10% weight loss in the last 6 months or 7.5% weight loss in the last 3 months- intentional of unintentional weight loss

2. Hair thinning or hair loss

3. Frequent or recurring infections

4. Poor caloric intake

5. Mental confusion and disorientation

6. Loss of muscle mass/bony prominences

7. Delayed wound healing

8. Consistent feeling of satiety (feeling full)

9. Dry, cracked, or flaky skin

10. Brittle nails

Protein-Calorie Malnutrition

11. Reduced appetite changed over 3,6,9,12 months

12. Easy bruising/poor skin integrity

13. Cachexia/frail appearance/decreased MAC

14. Loss of appetite/anorexia/dysphagia

15. Low blood pressure

16. Irregular heart rate/bradycardia/orthostatic hypotension

17. Edema (swelling) in the limbs or abdomen

18. Weakness and fatigue, poor balance and stamina. Tires easily/debility

19. Sunken cheeks, abdomen, or Eyes/owl eyes

20. Itchy skin

Protein-Calorie Malnutrition

S: Patient suffered a non-injury fall.
O: Patient has decreased muscle mass r/t poor caloric intake.
A: Patient unable to ambulate from bed to bathroom.
P: Transport wheelchair ordered.

S: Patient c/o feeling dizzy and weak.
O: Patient transfers from chair to bed.
A: BMI of 13, Albumin of 2.3, and hypotensive.
P: Monitor BP and educate on resting between changing positions.

S: Patient is weak and c/o discomfort on lower back.
O: Patient has a dark red area on bony prominence.
A: Patient has Stage 1 ulcer on coccyx and malnourished.
P. Obtain wound care orders and encourage frequent small meals and fluids.

S: Patient states she has no energy and dizzy.
O: 5lb weight loss in the last month, BMI decreased from 17-16.
A: Patient has severe malnutrition.
P: Encourage high protein meal supplements. Review safety and fall precautions.

Senile Degeneration of the Brain

Paint the Picture

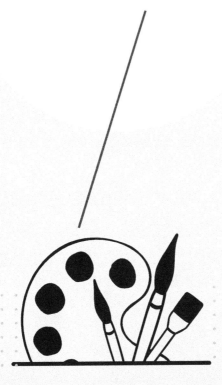

Senile Degeneration of the Brain

1. Severe fatigue and weakness-poor stamina and endurance, tires, easily

2. Disoriented/Low MMSE scale score (See Ch.5)

3. Difficulty communicating and speaking

4. Poor posture and balance/bed-bound

5. Inability to perform activities of daily living

6. Incontinence of bowel and bladder

7. Easily agitated and restless

8. Trouble swallowing/dysphagia/aspirating

9. Weight loss and decreased appetite

10. Sleep disturbances/insomnia

Senile Degeneration
of the Brain

11. Risk or history of recurring infections

12. Loss of any personal interests

13. Decreased responsiveness to stimuli

14. Changes in mood, such as depression or anxiety

15. Use of assistive devices-Broda chair, wheel chair, cushions, heel protectors, etc.

16. Forgetfulness and confusion

17. Encephalopathy (can also be a hospice primary dx)

18. Malnutrition (Chapter 4)

19. Poor mobility

20. Lack of interactions with others

Senile Degeneration
of the Brain

S: Patient is agitated and trying to get out of bed.
O: Patient is disoriented to time/place.
A: Patient is a fall risk, agitated, and confused.
P: Administer PRN Ativan. Review fall and safety precautions with caregiver.

S: Staff reports no BM in two days and poor fluid intake.
O: Dry mucous membranes. Skin tenting and dry.
A: Patient has s/sx of dehydration.
P: Encourage fluids if possible, Monitor I&O, review s/sx of decline.

S: Patient found in bed soiled from urine.
O: Spouse is unable to provide peri care with the patient in bed. Patient has been bedbound for two weeks.
A: Increased urinary incontinence and decreased mobility.
P: Obtain order for catheter placement and provide catheter care education to spouse.

S. Patient is not responding to husband when he speaks to her.
O: Spouse is tearful and having trouble coping/patient is withdrawn.
A: Patient is failing to thrive/ loss of interactions.
P: Education regarding disease process and referral for support services for spouse.

Atherosclerosis

Paint the Picture

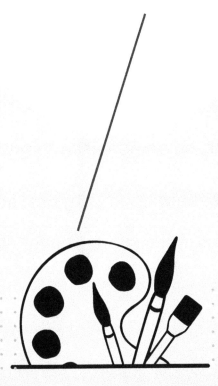

Atherosclerosis

1. Severe or uncontrolled angina or chest pain

2. Shortness of breath at rest or with exertion

3. Leg pain or cramping at rest or after walking.

4. Edema/ fluid retention

5. Coldness in extremities

6. Sores or wounds that are slow healing

7. Poor circulation in all extremities

8. Changes in vision

9. Confusion or increased forgetfulness

10. Fatigue with any physical activity

Atherosclerosis

11. Poor gait/hx of falls

12. Numbness and/or tingly in extremities

13. Irregular heartbeat and/or heart arrhythmias

14. History of heart attacks

15. Kidney failure or disease

16. Poor liver function

17. Weight loss

18. Hx of cardiac stents

19. Decreased ability to perform ADL's

20. Pacemaker with or without defibrillator

Atherosclerosis

S: Patient reports a painful wound on RLE.
O: Patient has a poor-healing pressure ulcer on RLE.
A: Circulation is poor in bilateral lower extremities. Wound measures 2inx1.5inx0.5in.
P: Education provided regarding smoke cessation. Wound care orders received.

S: Patient reports feelings of numbness in LLE.
O: LLE is red in color, cool to the touch, with 1+ edema.
A: Patient has s/sx of poor circulation with signs of fluid retention.
P: Patient encouraged to elevate BLE. Compression hose ordered.

S: Patient reports chest pain.
O: Spouse administers two doses of PRN Nitroglycerin.
A: Patient reports pain level of 5/10 after first dose and 0/10 after 2nd dose.
P: Education provided regarding s/sx of end stage. Atherosclerosis. Explained that it's common to have a decreased response to medications and a reminder regarding proper storage for medication.

Neurological Disorder

Paint the Picture

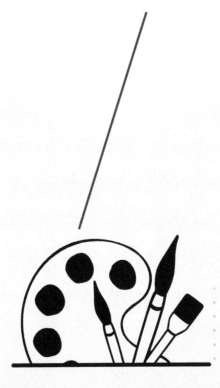

Neurological Disorder

Encephalopathy, Multiple Sclerosis,ALS, Lewy Body,....

1. Muscle weakness/Loss of sensation or numbness

2. Tremors or involuntary shaking movements

3. Hx of Seizures or convulsions

4. Recurring infections

5. Difficulty with coordination or balance

6. Difficulty swallowing/dysphagia

7. Vision problems, such as double vision or blindness

8. Hearing loss or ringing in the ears

9. Loss of bladder or bowel control

10. Chronic pain

Neurological Disorder

11. Extreme fatigue or weakness

12. Headaches or migraines

13. Sleep disturbances

14. Breathing difficulties

15. Changes in blood pressure or heart rate

16. Difficulty speaking

17. Paralysis

18. Risk for skin breakdown

19. Dependency of others for ADL's

20. Increase oral secretions/drooling

Neurological Disorder

S: The patient reports loss of urinary control.
O: Patient is incontinent of urine.
A: Increased urinary incontinence at night.
P: Review s/sx of Neurological Disease process, review proper skin and peri-care, encourage use of briefs at night.

S: Patient has left-sided paralysis.
O: Patient remains in the same position while in bed.
A: Patient unable to move left leg without assistance from others.
P: Prop extremities with pillows and educate caregiver on changing positions q 2 hours.

S: Spouse reports increased drooling when patient attempts to speak.
O: Excessive saliva noted while communicating with the patient.
A: Uncontrollable oral saliva/secretions.
P: Encourage use of a clothing protector and administer PRN medication for increased oral secretions.

05

Charting Tools

05

Patient Visit Note

Patient Name: _____

Diagnosis: _____

Date: _____

Start & End time: _____

Cert Period: _____

Caregiver or Facility: _____

Pain level: 0 1 2 3 4 5 6 7 8 9 10   Pain medication:

Vitals: <u>BP   P   T   R   O2</u>   Oxygen LPM:

PPS, NYHA, and/or FAST score: _____

MAC, Weight, or BMI: _____

Alert & Orient/Speech: _____

ADL's dependence: _____

Assistive Device Usage/Transfer: _____

DME: _____

Pertinent Labs: _____

Intake and Output: _____   Bowel Regimen: _____

Infections: _____

Incidents/Falls: _____

Wounds: _____

Other: _____

EXAMPLES OF COMPARATIVE DATA!!!

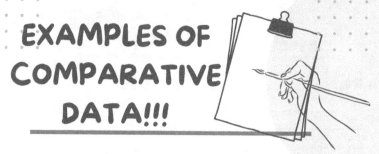

- Three months ago, the patient was able to walk 40 feet with a walker from living room to kitchen and back. She is now SOA when ambulating and takes a break every 20 feet.

- Currently sleeping 18-22 hours per day. Three months ago, the patient slept up to 14 hours in a 24-hour period.

- Over the last four months, dressing his upper and lower body has taken the patient up to two hours. He seldomly requires assistance with his pants. Six months ago, he was able to dress himself completely in one hour without assistance.

- Lasix increased 30 days ago from 20mg PO QD to 40mg PO QD to manage fluid retention.

- Spouse has managed medications for the last three months, setting up his weekly pill organizer. Six months ago, the patient was able to set up a weekly pill box without assistance from others.

- Nine months ago, patient used supplemental oxygen 3LPM via NC at night. Patient now uses supplemental oxygen at 4LPM continuously.

1. Spiritual and emotional support to patients and families

2. Conduct spiritual assessments

3. Provide end of life counseling

4. Create a care plan that meets spiritiual goals

5. Create a care plan that meets spiritual practices

6. Lead family group sessions

7. Listen to concerns and provide support

8. Inform IDT of any spiritual rituals

9. Team up with patient and family church

10. Assist with end of life services

11. Conduct Funeral services

12. Offer bereavement services

13. Offer spiritual support to hospice staff

14. Offer community support groups and additional resources

15. Advocate patient spiritual practices

Hospice Nurse Basics

1. Provide emotional support to patients and families

2. Community resources-food banks, support groups, volunteers, etc.

3. Mobile meal delivery services

4. Caregiver/ private duty services

5. Assist with Adult Daycare services

6. Lead family group sessions and offer support

7. Assist with medical transportation needs

8. Inform patient and family of VA Benefits

9. Assist with government programs-Medicaid, Medicare, TANF

10. Assist with planning documents- living will, advance directives, power of attorney, etc.

11. Financial Assistance-tax prep, utility/rent assistance, local church assistance

12. Offer bereavement services

13. Offer support to hospice staff

14. Offer community support groups and additional resources-council of aging

15. Assist with Emergency Response systems-life alert, smoke/ carbon monoxide alarms, utility company notifications of high risk patients

Hospice Nurse Basics

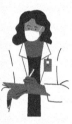

Hospice vs Palliative Care

- 6 months or less prognosis
- No fix or cure
- No aggressive treatment
- Focus is receiving EOL care that ensures QOL
- 24 on Call/ and standard visits as often as needed
- Medicare/ Medicaid or PI

- Terminal/Life limiting illnesses
- Symptom management
- Monitors changes in patient's health condition and keeps physician(s) informed
- Support and resources for patient&family
- Improve QOL

- Life limiting-Anytime during the illness
- Seeks aggressive treatment
- Continues to see specialists
- Focus is to maintain QOL while being aggressive
- No on call visits- monthly and prn visits
- Medicare/Medicaid or PI with copay

Hospice   ## Palliative

*Private Insurance=PI

Hospice Nurse Basics

95.

My personal breakdown
of the PPS SCALE

70%=ambulates with cane, or holds onto furniture and able to perform most ADLs

60%=walker PRN or full-time and minimally assisted with ADls

50%=walker or wheel chair, moderately assisted with ADLS

40%=chair/bed bound or uses assistive devices full-time, mainly assisted with ADLs

30%=bed bound, fully dependent on others for all ADLS. Eats small portions

20%= Significant decline, non ambulatory/non-transferable, fully dependent on others, little to no caloric intake

10%=Actively dying, fully dependent on others. No longer eating/NPO

0%=Death
Confusion and food intake changes can be seen at any percentage

Ulcer Scale

Guidelines for Staging of Pressure Ulcers*

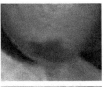

DEEP TISSUE INJURY

Purple or maroon localized area of discolored intact skin or blood-filled blister due to damage of underlying soft tissue from pressure and/or shear. The area may be preceded by tissue that is painful, firm, mushy, boggy, warmer or cooler as compared to adjacent tissue. Deep tissue injury may be difficult to detect in individuals with dark skin tones. Evolution may include a thin blister over a dark wound bed. The wound may further evolve and become covered by thin eschar. Evolution may be rapid exposing additional layers of tissue even with optimal treatment.

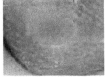

STAGE I

Intact skin with non-blanchable redness of a localized area usually over a bony prominence. Darkly pigmented skin may not have visible blanching; its color may differ from the surrounding area. The area may be painful, firm, soft, warmer or cooler as compared to adjacent tissue.

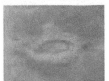

STAGE II

Partial thickness loss of dermis presenting as a shallow open ulcer with a red pink wound bed, without slough. May also present as an intact or open/ruptured serum-filled or sero-sanginous filled blister. Presents as a shiny or dry shallow ulcer without slough or bruising.**

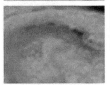

STAGE III

Full thickness tissue loss. Subcutaneous fat may be visible but bone, tendon or muscle are not exposed. Slough may be present but does not obscure the depth of tissue loss. May include undermining and tunneling. The depth of a Stage III pressure ulcer varies by anatomical location.

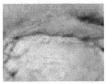

STAGE IV

Full thickness tissue loss with exposed bone, tendon or muscle. Slough or eschar may be present on some parts of the wound bed. Often include(s) undermining and tunneling. The depth of a Stage IV pressure ulcer varies by anatomical location.

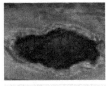

UNSTAGEABLE

Full thickness tissue loss in which the base of the ulcer is covered by slough (yellow, tan, gray, green or brown) and/or eschar (tan, brown or black) in the wound bed.

WOUND ASSESSMENT CHECKLIST

- Location
- Size
- Dressing Used

- Stage
- Pressure Redistribution
- Nutritional Assessment

- Drainage (Amount/Color/Odor)
- Viable Tissue in Wound
- Undermining/Tunneling

*National Pressure Ulcer Advisory Panel (NPUAP) - Accessed November 2014. **Bruising indicates deep tissue injury.

BMI Calculator

WEIGHT	lbs	90	100	110	120	130	140	150	160	170	180	190	200	210	220	230	240	250	260	270	280
	kgs	41	45	50	54	59	64	68	73	77	82	86	91	95	100	104	109	113	118	122	127
HEIGHT		Underweight					Healthy					Overweight				Obese				Extremely Obese	
ft/in	cm																				
4'8"	142.2	20	22	25	27	29	31	34	36	38											
4'9"	144.7	19	22	24	26	28	30	32	35	37	39										
4'10"	147.3	19	21	23	25	27	29	31	33	36	38										
4'11"	149.8	18	20	22	24	26	28	30	32	34	36	38									
4'12"	152.4	18	20	21	23	25	27	29	31	33	35	37	39								
5'1"	154.9	17	19	21	23	25	26	28	30	32	34	36	38								
5'2"	157.4	16	18	20	22	24	26	27	29	31	33	35	37	38							
5'3"	160.0	16	18	19	21	23	25	27	28	30	32	34	35	37	39						
5'4"	162.5	15	17	19	21	22	24	26	27	29	31	33	34	36	38	39					
5'5"	165.1	15	17	18	20	22	23	25	27	28	30	32	33	35	37	38					
5'6"	167.6	15	16	18	19	21	23	24	26	27	29	31	32	34	36	37	39				
5'7"	170.1	14	16	17	19	20	22	24	25	27	28	30	31	33	34	36	38	39			
5'8"	172.7	14	15	17	18	20	21	23	24	26	27	29	30	32	33	35	37	38			
5'9"	175.2	13	15	16	18	19	21	22	24	25	27	28	30	31	33	34	35	37	38		
5'10"	177.8	13	14	16	17	19	20	22	23	24	26	27	29	30	32	33	34	36	37	39	
5'11"	180.3	13	14	15	17	18	20	21	22	24	25	27	28	29	31	32	33	35	36	38	39
6'0"	182.8	12	14	15	16	18	19	20	22	23	24	26	27	28	30	31	33	34	35	37	38
6'1"	185.4	12	13	15	16	17	18	20	21	22	24	25	26	28	29	30	32	33	34	36	37
6'2"	187.9	12	13	14	15	17	18	19	21	22	23	24	26	27	28	30	31	32	33	35	36
6'3"	190.5	11	13	14	15	16	18	19	20	21	23	24	25	26	28	29	30	31	33	34	35
6'4"	193.0	11	12	13	15	16	17	18	19	21	22	23	24	26	27	28	29	30	32	33	34
6'5"	195.5	11	12	13	14	15	17	18	19	20	21	23	24	25	26	27	28	30	31	32	33
6'6"	198.1	10	12	13	14	15	16	17	18	20	21	22	23	24	25	27	28	29	30	31	32
6'7"	200.6	10	11	12	14	15	16	17	18	19	20	21	23	24	25	26	27	28	29	30	32
6'8"	203.2	10	11	12	13	14	15	16	18	19	20	21	22	23	24	25	26	27	29	30	31
6'9"	205.7	10	11	12	13	14	15	16	17	18	19	20	21	23	24	25	26	27	28	29	30
6'10"	208.2	9	10	12	13	14	15	16	17	18	19	20	21	22	23	24	25	26	27	28	29
6'11"	210.8	9	10	11	12	13	14	15	16	17	18	19	20	21	22	23	25	26	27	28	29

MMSE Scale

MINI MENTAL STATE EXAMINATION (MMSE)

| Name: |
| DOB: |
| Hospital Number: |

One point for each answer   **DATE:**

ORIENTATION Year Season Month Date Time	....../ 5	....../ 5	....../ 5
Country Town District Hospital Ward/Floor	....../ 5	....../ 5	....../ 5
REGISTRATION Examiner names three objects (e.g. apple, table, penny) and asks the patient to repeat (1 point for each correct. THEN the patient learns the 3 names repeating until correct).	....../ 3	....../ 3	....../ 3
ATTENTION AND CALCULATION Subtract 7 from 100, then repeat from result. Continue five times: 100, 93, 86, 79, 65. (Alternative: spell "WORLD" backwards: DLROW).	....../ 5	....../ 5	....../ 5
RECALL Ask for the names of the three objects learned earlier.	....../ 3	....../ 3	....../ 3
LANGUAGE Name two objects (e.g. pen, watch).	....../ 2	....../ 2	....../ 2
Repeat "No ifs, ands, or buts".	....../ 1	....../ 1	....../ 1
Give a three-stage command. Score 1 for each stage. (e.g. "Place index finger of right hand on your nose and then on your left ear").	....../ 3	....../ 3	....../ 3
Ask the patient to read and obey a written command on a piece of paper. The written instruction is: "Close your eyes".	....../ 1	....../ 1	....../ 1
Ask the patient to write a sentence. Score 1 if it is sensible and has a subject and a verb.	....../ 1	....../ 1	....../ 1

COPYING: Ask the patient to copy a pair of intersecting pentagons

	....../ 1	....../ 1	....../ 1

TOTAL: ....../ 30   ....../ 30   ....../ 30

MMSE scoring
24-30: no cognitive impairment
18-23: mild cognitive impairment
0-17: severe cognitive impairment

OME   Oxford Medical Education

FAST Scale

Functional Assessment Scale (FAST)

1	No difficulty either subjectively or objectively.
2	Complains of forgetting location of objects. Subjective work difficulties.
3	Decreased job functioning evident to co-workers. Difficulty in traveling to new locations. Decreased organizational capacity. *
4	Decreased ability to perform complex task, (e.g., planning dinner for guests, handling personal finances, such as forgetting to pay bills, etc.)
5	Requires assistance in choosing proper clothing to wear for the day, season or occasion, (e.g. pt may wear the same clothing repeatedly, unless super-vised.*
6	Occasionally or more frequently over the past weeks. * for the following **A)** Improperly putting on clothes without assistance or cueing . **B)** Unable to bathe properly (not able to choose proper water temp) **C)** Inability to handle mechanics of toileting (e.g., forget to flush the toilet, does not wipe properly or properly dispose of toilet tissue) **D)** Urinary incontinence **E)** Fecal incontinence
7	**A)** Ability to speak limited to approximately ≤ 6 intelligible different words in the course of an average day or in the course of an intensive interview. **B)** Speech ability is limited to the use of a single intelligible word in an average day or in the course of an intensive interview **C)** Ambulatory ability is lost (cannot walk without personal assistance.) **D)** Cannot sit up without assistance (e.g., the individual will fall over if there are not lateral rests [arms] on the chair.) **E)** Loss of ability to smile. **F)** Loss of ability to hold up head independently.

*Scored primarily on information obtained from a knowledgeable informant.

NYHA Functional Classification

I
No limitation of physical activity. Ordinary physical activity does not cause symptoms of HF

II
Slight limitation of physical activity. Comfortable at rest, but ordinary physical activity results in symptoms of HF.

III
Marked limitation of physical activity. Comfortable at rest, but less than ordinary activity causes symptoms of HF.

IV
Unable to carry on any physical activity without symptoms of HF, or symptoms of HF at rest.

1. Tense, rigid, guarded

2. Heavy breathing

3. Moan/groan/grunts

4. Restless behaviors

5. Crying /screaming

6. Irritability

7. Changes in blood pressure

8. Increased heart rate

9. Paleness or changes in skin

10. Grimace/frown

11. Repetitive movements

12. Guarded movements

13. Facial movements

14. Changes in sleep pattern

15. Aggression

Hospice Nurse Basics

8 Activities of Daily Living

1. Continence

2. Bathing

3. Eating/Swallowing

4. Feeding

5. Ambulating/Transfers

6. Memory

7. Dressing

8. Toileting

Hospice Nurse Basics

8 Instrumental Activities Of Daily Living

1. Prepare Meals

2. Manage Finances

3. Home Maintenance

4. Laundry/housekeeping

5. Shop

6. Use a telephone

7. Manage Medications

8. Drive/Transportation

Hospice Nurse Basics

Alternatives to Morphine

Hospice Formulary

Hydromorphone

Oxycodone

Fentanyl

Methadonee

@hospicenursebasics

S/SX of Declining and Dying

1. Non-responsive to stimulation

2. Little to no urine output or stool output

3. Not eating or drinking

4. Non-verbal/unintelligible speech pattern

5. Comatose state

6. Changes in vitals-Low oxygen saturation, Bp, Pulse

7. Changes in skin color

8. Change in body odor

9. Changes in breathing pattern

10. Blank stare/gloss or baby doll eyes

11. Reaching

12. Speaking to past loved ones. angels. etc.

13. Patient states they are passing away

14. Butterfly Ulcer

15. Ears pulled/pinned back

AND MANY MORE!!

Hospice Nurse Basics

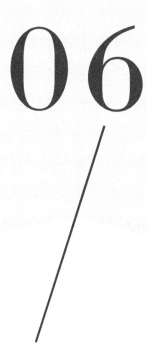

06

C H A P T E R
Conclusion

06

CONCLUSION:

REMEMBER you work 9-5 (give or take). Try not to get distracted by things that are not related to work during work hours, and if you are having trouble or have any concerns, speak to your Supervisor. Remember, closed mouths don't get fed. LOL!!!

I really hope you enjoyed this book.
I hope you find that you are able to have your work-life balance, cut your charting time in half, and become the EDUCATED AF HOSPICE NURSE for your team!

THE EDUCATED AF HOSPICE NURSE!!

**BY MAKHAELA WILLIAMS
HOSPICE NURSE BASICS**

HOSPICENURSEBASICS@GMAIL.COM

INDEX

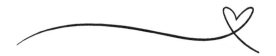

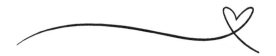

INDEX

INDEX

INDEX

INDEX

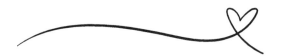

INDEX

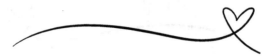

INDEX

INDEX

REFERENCES

1. Pin by Sally Richards on Nursing ~ Palliative Care: Elderly care, Hospice nurse, Elderly caregiver
https://www.pinterest.co.uk/pin/21399141978177330
3/ext

2. https://co.pinterest.com/pin/77124212360480809/

3. Mini-mental state examination (MMSE) - Oxford Medical Education: Medical education, Mental, Preschool writing
https://www.pinterest.at/pin/69665125474468430/ittle bit of body text

4. New York Heart Association (NYHA) Classification - severity of HF🖤🖤 -------------...: Emergency medicine, Hospice nurse, Psychiatric mental health nursing
https://www.pinterest.com/pin/40813940361683122/

5. Pressure ulcer staging ...: Home health nurse, Wound care nursing, Wound care
https://www.pinterest.com/pin/128493395619058201/

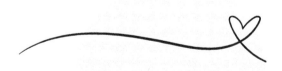

hospicenursebasics@gmail.com

BY MAKHAELA WILLIAMS
HOSPICE NURSE BASICS

REFERENCES

Check out the HOSPICE NURSE BASICS Free Hospice VS Palliative Care Kahoot game to play with your staff!!!

FOLLOW US ON **YOUTUBE** AND **TIKTOK** @ HOSPICENURSEBASCIS

Reach me via email at: hospicenursebasics@gmail.com

**BY MAKHAELA WILLIAMS
HOSPICE NURSE BASICS**

NOTES

NOTES

♥

NOTES

♥